The Colon Cancer

Diet

Dr. Christopher Maloney, N.D.

DEDICATION

To all of you, who are dealing with the fear and uncertainty
of colon cancer. May you find healing.

CONTENTS

ACKNOWLEDGMENTS

I want to thank every member of my medical team. They did a wonderful job, and while I will poke fun at them throughout these pages I am truly thankful. I would like to thank Lisa and Pam, who read through the book for me and make invaluable changes. I would also like to thank my family, my friends and patients for being there with love, support and fruit salads. There are not words enough to thank my wife.

WARNING:

The following book is for informational use only. Please discuss it with your loved ones, your caregivers, and your doctors. I am happy to provide the studies used in this text, but omitted them for ease in viewing. Medicine is constantly changing, and new studies may have already come out that contradict what is written here. Please email me or have your doctors email me for studies and information at: docmaloneynd@gmail.com. The studies are also available online at: naturopathicmaine.com

Preface To The Second Edition

Thank you to all of you who have written to me about your own cancer journeys! As I progress myself, I've had ups and downs. The publication of the first edition of this book was rushed because my labs were getting worse and I was concerned that I had metastasis.

But since then I've had a clean colonoscopy and better labs. So life is looking up. I feel incredibly lucky and my heart goes out to all of you starting this journey.

I've gone through the medical literature again for this edition, and tried to expand on what we know will help. We're just starting to see big studies being started in this area, so I'm hopeful some of you will get to participate and benefit.

Please, if you have conflicting information, particularly studies, I'd love to see it. The beauty of modern publication is that I can improve my work for you.

-Chris Maloney, May 2017

1 Who Needs This Book?

I did. When I was diagnosed in November of 2015 with colon cancer, I went looking for this book. Given the avalanche of diet books, I figured someone had written one for me. No luck. So I set out to find out what I should be eating as a newly diagnosed colon cancer patient, and ended up creating what I needed.

You need this book if you or someone you love is dealing with the terror of colon cancer. Unless the entire medical model has shifted since this book was published, you won't find anything like it written by someone who is both a patient and a doctor.

If you have a history of colon cancer in your family you need this book. We have been told family history matters more and diet and lifestyle matter less than they really do.

I wrote this book to provide a framework for those of us

who have been diagnosed with colon cancer who are trying to live as best we can between blood work, lab tests, and doctors' visits. With you in mind I made it short, sweet, and hopefully a little funny because God knows we could use a laugh.

What makes me qualified to write this book? For over a decade before I got my diagnosis I'd been in family practice, working with patients who didn't fit the conventional medical model. These are people who are told to live with it or to go home and get their affairs in order. So I'd seen my share of metastatic cancer patients. And no, I didn't magically cure anyone, though several cured themselves. I can't take credit for someone else's miracle. As a Naturopathic doctor of last resort, I was very conservative and didn't make crazy promises or promote extreme treatments.

I saved the extreme treatments for my personal life. When I tried something like weight loss, I tried everything. Every diet under the sun. They all worked short term. Extreme measures can be effective and they get old quickly. I'd soon "fall off the wagon" and regain the weight.

But when I got colon cancer, all the weight just dropped off me. It has stayed away far more easily than ever before. I've got this motivation program I call "the screaming fear of death" that really helps me keep the pounds off. Be careful what you wish for.

Given my background as someone who regularly sees

"incurable" patients and tries to come up with treatments, I spend far more time researching than is healthy. Since my diagnosis I've cut down my hours at the computer, but I still have a knack for finding things well after others would have thrown in the towel. So, while you could spend well over a hundred hours yourself looking up everything, I can save you time by explaining the studies in English rather than medicalese.

If you count in all the years I spent learning medicalese (which is like Chinese but more boring) so I could translate for you, then this book is a real bargain.

My hope is that by the time you finish reading these few pages you'll know what you can do to help yourself and those you love live longer with a diagnosis of colon cancer, as well as what you can tell your family to help them avoid it.

2 Finding The Colon Cancer Diet

When I started doing my research for this book, I learned that we know a great deal about colon cancer. Well, we know a great deal about how to perform surgery on patients with colon cancer.

Most of the studies on colon cancer in the last ten years have been a discussion about whether cutting someone wide open or using little cuts (laparoscopic) in surgery is better. Laparoscopic wins, but mostly because surgeons usually only open someone up when things start to go south (tearing, bleeding, you get the idea). So it would be fairer to say that getting open surgery means you have more cancer, not that the open surgery itself is worse for you.

We also know a great deal about what causes colon cancer in the general population. It turns out that our standard western diet and lifestyle (sitting all the time) are the perfect breeding grounds for colon cancer. The increased risk from a poor lifestyle is very high.

So, yes, you probably contributed to your colon cancer's growth (unless you have a rare genetic cause). Notice I said contributed, not caused. You may have helped it grow, but you didn't cause it (we'll deal with the emotional impact of that fear later).

If anyone tells you that you caused your cancer, slap them for me. But also slap anyone who says you should ignore your diet and lifestyle's contribution to your cancer's cause (just bad luck). Looking for the contributing causes in your life can help you improve your chances of staying healthy going forward.

I wrote this book for those of you in waiting mode, like me. If you are currently in chemo or getting radiated, chances are the best thing you can do is get in as many of the right kind of calories as you can. I'll give some suggestions, but I also forgive you ahead of time if all you feel like doing is lying around and eating Ho-Hos. Forgive yourself. You are undergoing the equivalent of an internal war. Keeping your morale and your energy up is the first priority. If this book helps you, keep reading. If it annoys you, throw it halfway across the room (with those chemo-weakened arms) and leave it lying there until you feel better.

We're going to take a quick tour through the genetics of colon cancer, talk about diet and exercise (hint: they do matter) and also talk about some "supplements" (including aspirin and coffee). I'll cover a couple of the well-known alternative diets (Gerson and Mediterranean). We'll talk about them in terms of colon cancer risk.

I'll also give you my own diet choices. I'm doing far more to stay well than I would recommend for others based on what we know for certain from the studies we have on colon cancer and diet. We'll end on the meaning and focus you give your cancer. Come on, doesn't every diet book end with a "lifetime" chapter where the author tells you it's going to be easy to do this for the rest of your life? It won't be easy, but we can get there.

3 Does It Run In Your Family?

"Does it run in your family?" is the first question I get after being diagnosed with colon cancer at early age of forty-five. It never fails. "Run?" I want to say, "it practically gallops." But that wouldn't be true. My family history is disturbingly clean.

You would think that the doctors would know better by now. The family history question should only come up after a long discussion of lifestyle issues. But my local cancer center seems desperate for my complete family tree to track down "where on earth my cancer came from."

We know where it came from. It came from where almost all colon cancers come from: diet and lifestyle. But we're going to talk about genetics first to get that out of the way.

The "runs in your family" question assumes that if you have

a family member with colon cancer, you are more likely to get colon cancer yourself. And it's true, you are. But you're not as likely to get it as you'd think.

For those of you who've had a colonoscopy, you know there's cancer and there's polyps. Polyps are like the moles of the gut, little bits of gut tissue sticking out from the walls of your intestines. They look something like skin tags on your skin, only fatter at the base. You can have lots of polyps and no cancer. But the more polyps, the greater the risk one of them could turn into cancer.

A lot of what we know about family colon cancer risk concerns polyps, not cancer. Remember, polyps aren't cancer, they just increase your risk of getting cancer. If you have a close family member who has a lot of polyps, you double your chances of also having polyps. If you have two close family members with polyps, the risk doubles again. If they have large polyps, then you have double the risk of having large polyps. Remember, again, polyps are not cancer. But you do share your chances of getting lots of polyps with your family.

Twice or even four times the risk (two or more relatives) sounds like a huge risk if it runs in your family. But remember, that's just the risk for polyps. The risk of actual cancer is much lower.

How low is the actual cancer risk from your family history? Let's start with an average fifty-year-old guy (sorry ladies, we get more colon cancer), call him John. John and ninety-nine of his closest buddies go in for colonoscopies together. I don't know, maybe it's an Elks Club fundraiser and they do it every five years. Of the hundred guys in the colonoscopy fundraising crowd, two of them will show up with colon cancer some time in their lives. That means John has a very, very good chance of never getting colon cancer.

But John changes Elks Club lodges. In his new Elks Club Lodge with one hundred members, everybody has a close relative (mom, dad, sister, not cousin) with colon cancer. These guys are very motivated and do their colonoscopies every three years. At some point in their lives, four of them will show up with colon cancer. That means John still has a really, really good chance of never getting colon cancer even though it doubled when his mom was diagnosed.

John changes Elks Club Lodges again. Now all these one hundred new guys have two family members with colon cancer. They are very, very motivated, and they go in for their colonoscopies every year. It's a big fundraiser. Even though they all have two family members with colon cancer, only seven of the hundred Elks Club members will ever come down with colon cancer in their lifetimes.

As John has progressed up through the Elks Lodges and increased his own risk of getting colon cancer, he still has a greater than ninety percent chance of never getting colon cancer in his lifetime. And that's with a mom and a sister who have been diagnosed with it.

So for most of us, having a second-cousin or a great-aunt with colon cancer (in my case a great-grandmother) isn't really increasing our risk of developing colon cancer. It's scary and it should make us watchful, but not that worried.

Now let's do a mean thing to our friend John. Some members of his medical team suspect John is part of one of those unlucky families that are really at high risk of getting colon cancer. His doctor tells him that, while only five percent of colon cancers have been proven to come directly from family genetics, he thinks that John's family is part of that five percent. He thinks John's family has Lynch Syndrome.

Lynch Syndrome folks inherit mismatched repair genes, so their bodies don't do well fighting cancers. If John had known earlier, he would have gotten lots of colonoscopies starting at twenty-five, and his sister would have had her ovaries and uterus tested for cancers as well. If John and his ninety-nine Elks' Lodge pals all had Lynch Syndrome, almost eighty of them would have come down with colon cancer in their lifetimes. But the Lodge would have had to recruit far and wide, because Lynch Syndrome is very rare.

Now, John gets good news because he comes back negative for Lynch Syndrome. He doesn't have that problem in his genes. But his doctor is now convinced John has another genetic disease that causes colon cancer, familial polyposis.

Familial polyposis folks grow polyps the way dandelions grow on an organic lawn. What's the treatment? Cut it out! Cut it all out! All of the colon must go, pretty much before the family member can finish puberty.

Many familial polyposis patients have their colons removed before they reach their eighteenth birthdays. Even years later only about half of them have continence (can hold their stool) which tends to bring down their quality of life, but beats the heck out of dying. I can't imagine the psychological effects of telling a ten-year-old they might die of colon cancer unless they have their bowel taken out before they're old enough to vote. And having the colon out may not be the end of their cancer risk, as familial polyposis families also get far more thyroid cancer

Fortunately for most of us, the number of families with familial polyposis is very, very low. At fifty, John is extremely unlikely to have familial polyposis without anyone else in his family having discovered it yet (less chance than a lightning strike on his head giving him a sudden hair growth).

If you don't have familial polyposis and your family doesn't have Lynch Syndrome, how concerned should you be about your family history of colon cancer? A lot less than you'd expect. Despite the immediate urge to get everyone in a new patient's family tested, they aren't at that much greater risk from your genes, and may be at a greater risk for colon cancer from your shared diet and lifestyle.

So why the focus on family history? The medical reality is that if colon cancer metastasizes we don't have great outcomes, so we need to catch it early. The "family history" angle is meant to bring more patients in for testing. Right now medical researchers are looking for other families like Lynch Syndrome families to see if they can target more high risk people before they fall ill.

Clarifying those few families at highest risk for colon cancer really helps them, but the focus on family history may lull those without a family history into a false sense of security. People may have rectal bleeding for years and not get checked because they don't have a family history of colon cancer. Overestimating the family connection can act as a "buffer" excuse, allowing those without the history to keep the fear of colon cancer (and testing) at bay.

For those of us on the other side of the colon cancer diagnosis, it's good to know that a family history isn't as terrible a burden on our loved ones as we'd expect from colon cancer ads. We haven't doomed our relatives to our fate because of our genetics, so take a moment to let go of that particular cancer-related guilt. And yes, they should still get tested and be more careful with their lifestyles.

4 What Causes 95% of Colon Cancer?

The doctor trying to diagnose John as being in a high-risk colon cancer family mentions that only five percent of cancers are solely caused by genetics. That means 95% of colon cancers are caused by something else. As best we can tell, almost all colon cancers are caused by diet and lifestyle.

There may be some overlap. Even though Elks' Lodge John doesn't have a direct genetic cause, the genes he inherited may make him more reactive to diet and lifestyle triggers for colon cancer growth. John's gut may get inflamed easily, leading to more polyps and a higher risk of cancer. Think of it in the same way that being fair skinned doesn't mean you get skin cancer, but does make you more likely to burn. John's gut may "sunburn" easily from the wrong foods sitting in his colon all day.

A number of families may have both genetics and diet/lifestyle working against them. Almost a quarter of people coming down with colon cancer have a close family history, so those people could all have some genetic weakness that sets them up for colon cancer. But so far, when we're looking for a direct link, only about five percent have the "dad got it, I'll get it" genetic direct cause. The rest are considered to have a combined contribution from both lifestyle and genetics.

Someone not wanting to do diet and lifestyle changes could say that all those people with a family history are all genetic. They have the genes, we just haven't isolated out which genes yet. So we shouldn't consider them, and the title of this chapter is wrong.

Let's assume for the moment that every single person with a family history of colon cancer will eventually be found with a completely genetic cause. None of them could benefit from any diet or lifestyle changes. That still leaves three-quarters of colon cancer patients as "spontaneous." No family history, and still came down with colon cancer.

So, let's join John and his ninety-nine buddies in his new lodge where they've all come down with colon cancer. (This Elks Lodge is a terrible one to belong to. What are they feeding these guys?) John is surprised to find that of all the Lodge members, only twenty-five of them have a family history. And only five of them have an absolute, "dad had this, I got this" genetic history. That leaves seventy-five guys sitting around the Lodge wondering what the heck happened. John's got the family history, but he doesn't have an absolute genetic link that his doctors could find. So he might or might not be able to blame his genes. If he was a betting man, he might bet on something else besides his genetics given that most of the people in the room don't have any genetic cause at all.

Most of the guys in the room full of colon cancer folks are old, older than John. Colon cancer used to be an old person's disease. The average age of diagnosis is still in a person's seventies. But we're seeing more and more younger and younger patients with colon cancer. The genetics haven't been changing, but the diet and lifestyle of younger people has been.

The connection between what we eat and colon cancer hasn't entered into the medical framework for treating colon cancer. Not once during my entire treatment, from colonoscopy through follow up, did anyone advise me to permanently change my diet.

For a colon cancer doctor, the goal is rapid intervention, and something like diet isn't considered rapid enough even if we knew exactly what you should eat. Given limited time, a cancer doctor is going to spend it talking about a chemotherapy or a second surgery that she believes is going to make a quicker difference in the disease progress. She also assumes that patients will be resistant to diet changes, even if it might dramatically improve their outcomes. Why would doctors spend time explaining something that doesn't work as fast and that their patients are not likely to do? But, even though we're resistant to change, colon cancer patients should at least have an idea of what they can do to help themselves.

5 What To Avoid

So what causes colon cancer in most people if it's not genetics? We have a pretty good idea. Turns out that the tons of food you run through your colon every year affects how well your colon repairs itself and how likely it is to start getting cancerous.

It's not that complicated an idea. Cancer is cell growth that gets out of control in response to a lifetime of irritation from trauma or chemicals. If you rubbed your elbow with sandpaper and dunked it in chemicals for twenty years, chances are you'd develop some strange cell growth on your elbow (and should probably get your head checked, you lunatic). Over time, a few of those cells might become cancerous. So if you dowse your lower gut with day glow chemicals and old meat in a perpetual alcohol and sugar bath, you can also increase your cancer risk over a lifetime.

We feed poor mice a standard Western diet and they develop colon cancer at much higher rates. The same thing happens to humans when we track diet choices across different cultures. But since we don't have large laboratories where human volunteers in cages are force fed fast food, the human results are still considered "preliminary." A cautious person might still want to avoid eating a standard Western diet to lower his or her risk of colon cancer.

Ah, but you and I already have colon cancer. Does it really matter what we eat now? Isn't the damage already done? No. Humans diagnosed with colon cancer who continue on the standard western diet still have the same risks and the same issues. Poor eaters with colon cancer had three times the rate of cancer recurrence. Time to take evasive action!

In the world of cancer doctors, diet is a bad word. Other than cleaning your bowel out for surgery, they don't care what you put into it. On discharge, my very-forward thinking and research-oriented hospital nurse told me that I could go right back to my regular diet. Her suggestion was for me to get a Denny's Grand Slam, which has to be the colon cancer diet equivalent of giving a lung cancer patient a pack of cigarettes.

Two days earlier I'd had my bowels torn open, sectioned out, and stapled together. But now I was being set loose into the world of fast food. Heck, if I'd been a closet drinker, this was my opportunity to get that buzz you only get after your stomach has been empty for five days.

Can I just say you want to ignore that joke and reverse coming out of surgery exactly the same way you went in? You want to eat really good food, mostly soups, broths, and soft things, until it doesn't hurt every time you move. Anything else is just loco. I don't have a study for loco, you can just find out the hard way if you'd like.

My nurse cautioned me this way, "if you get the Denny's Grand Slam, you can eat it. But you probably won't eat that much of it at first because your stomach is so small." Duly noted. And in passing let me say again that a Denny's Grand Slam pretty much embodies exactly what you shouldn't eat if you want to avoid a second trip to "chop-out-a-piece-of-my-gut" central. Imagine handing a guy who's just had a lung out from lung cancer a pack of cigarettes and telling him to smoke in moderation at first because he only has one lung now.

At this point, a few of you might know that there's a possible link between processed meat and colon cancer. As my oncologist said, "it's not hard data" because it's based on population studies and stuffing mice full of nasty old jerky until they get cancer.

We don't have any studies on force feeding human volunteers Slim Jims until they form tumors. So we can't say for certain that it causes colon cancer.

We don't have any large labs somewhere in Nebraska where volunteers sit around in cages. So we're going to be talking about people doing surveys of diet or doing bad things to small animals when we talk about diet and colon cancer. No one can "prove" some part of your diet caused anything for you. We can just make our best guess that there might be a connection. Feel free to ignore it, but at least you have the information.

So what should we avoid?

Smoking

Lots of alcohol.

Lots of red meat.

Lots of processed meat.

Lots of fried meat.

Lots of grilled meat.

Lots of broiled meat.

Refined flour.

Sugar.

Sugar cane.

Sweets.

Desserts.

Hopefully, if you're paying attention, you'll notice a theme.

Sugar (including alcohol) and red meat. There's also a clear set of rules about how you shouldn't cook your meat. Now, I know the paleo-diet group will already be hedging, "they didn't study my grass-fed, organic pet cow who meditates. That meat is different." To which I say, prove it. (Having cancer means you don't always have time to be polite.) Please show me a study of people diagnosed with colon cancer who have less recurrence of that cancer after eating a lot of meat. Just compare them to those eating less meat or those just eating plants. Until I see the "Zen cow study" we've got nothing to talk about. What we have right now are studies that estimate I can triple (not just double) my risk of colon cancer recurrence by eating primarily from the list above. That's not something I want to ignore, even if it's not "hard data."

Let's go into a little more depth about what we should avoid.

Smoking. Less is better. Yes, smoking increases your risk of colon cancer recurrence, as well as causing about 20% of colon cancers. Current smokers with colon cancer tend to die slightly sooner than past smokers.

Alcohol. Drinking more increases your risk of liver metastases. There is no "safe" amount of alcohol for people with colon cancer.

Lots of red meat. If you are eating six servings of red meat a week and want to cut your risk from very high to very low, drop down to less than two servings a week. How much is a serving? About the size of your kid's smart phone.

Lots of processed meat. Don't eat six servings of processed meat a week. Cut it down to less than two servings to lower your risk of recurrence. All meats are included from here on.

Lots of fried meat. I think you're getting the idea. Six servings: bad. Less than two servings a week: good. Let's call this the six-to-two rule. Or Rule 62, which makes it sounds like we have our own lingo. Colon cancer patients can yell at each other, "How's Rule 62?" "Working on it, getting there." Wouldn't it be nice to have the doctors confused for a change?

Lots of grilled meat. Six bad. Two good.

Lots of broiled meat. Rule 62 applies. Who likes lots of broiled meat?

Remember, you don't get two servings of each kind of

meat! You get two servings of red meat a week, however you decide to cook it.

Refined flour. To drop your risk of recurrence, eat less than two servings a day. Those at the highest risk ate six servings a day, so now rule 62 applies to every day for refined flour.

Don't get confused. Drop your funky meat intake to less than two servings a <u>week</u>, and drop your refined flour intake to less than two servings a <u>day</u>. How big is a serving? A slice, a piece, a half-cup, again roughly the size of your kid's smart phone.

Sugar. Sugar cane. Sweets. Desserts. The number here is much lower than Rule 62. People at the highest risk of recurrence ate more than two desserts a day. The people at the lowest risk ate less than one.

Try to avoid getting your "dessert" sugar added invisibly to packaged goods, because by avoiding them you could possibly eat a dessert every other day. Again a dessert serving size is the size of your kid's smart phone, which must be looking pretty tasty by this point. Do they make them in meat flavor? How about a lollipop case?

Now, I know for myself that I wanted the "rules" about exactly what I could eat (so I could break them). Before any of you write to me and ask what the exact rules are about eating a piece of baked -but reheated in the microwave- piece of organic Zen pork, let me be clear. We are talking about the rest of your life.

None of us will be perfect for the rest of our lives. We will all fall off the wagon. So before you start beating your brother-in-law because his "vegan" beans contained bacon ("Are you trying to kill me?") take a moment. Remember the lifetime dietary rule, which says you want to do something most of the time and not get sidetracked by occasional falls off the wagon into a barbeque pit. Just get right back on, and don't worry about it. If it starts happening daily, well, you've decided to roll your dice with the extra risk. It's your life.

6 What To Eat

Now things get really interesting. It's easy to say what not to eat, it's a lot harder to say what you should eat once you've been diagnosed with colon cancer.

I know there are a million people out there telling you what to eat to cure cancer. Many of them have really good stories about people who did their diets and cured cancer. But surprisingly few of them have studies done that show their diet cures cancer for everyone who tries it. Individual stories are great, but we don't see the other individual stories. These are the unhappy ones that start, "I did this diet perfectly and still died of cancer." Those are the stories that "true believers" on a specific diet don't want to hear.

Part of being a true believer in a particular diet is thinking only positive thoughts about your diet. If you question their "locusts and honey, living in a cave" diet they will get very angry. "It's right there in the bible!" they'll say. Or "Dr. Ijust Madethisup has three degrees in oncology. He can't be wrong!" Unfortunately, neither one of those beliefs will mean that you or I will live longer eating only tree frogs and pond scum (yum, pond scum).

We do know that avoiding a ton of red meat and straight sugar helps avoid colon cancer recurrence. That's a great start. We need to eat things other than red meat and sugar. It's part of the balanced five things that we know are helpful for colon cancer patients: good weight, exercise, not smoking, limiting alcohol, and a healthy diet.

But what's a healthy diet? When researchers compared patients who avoided the "bad" foods with patients who actively sought out "good" foods, avoidance won. The colon cancer patients who ate a "prudent" diet, a diet based on lots of fruits and vegetables, fish and bird meat, didn't do any better than people who just avoided eating lots of red meat and sugar.

One might ask what exactly the "avoiding" folks were eating since red meat, refined flour, and sugar weren't on the menu. Chances are that they also ate fruits and vegetables, fish and bird meat. They just didn't brag about it as much as the "prudent" crowd. But the prudent crowd's risk of recurrence didn't drop to zero like we would have hoped.

Now we must speculate on what a healthy diet could be. Since we don't have definitive studies, we need to look at some lesser studies and see what we can find. Remember that the largest studies are surveys and rat trials, so now we're clearly entering the "maybe" area of the medical literature.

One medical reviewer says all colon cancer patients (all cancer patients, everybody) should adapt the Mediterranean diet. If you missed the diet wars, the Mediterranean diet is one that focuses on good fats, fruits and vegetables, whole grains and nuts, with a little meat and sugar. Imagine a large homemade Italian dinner, using whole grain everything. A big salad, lots of olive oil, a choice of whole grains, maybe some meat in the tomato sauce.

We see less overall cancer in people who consume that traditional Mediterranean diet. But those Mediterranean people also have a very different way of living, so making the dietary recommendation may not be accurate. It's a little like looking at the Amish and concluding their whole grain diet makes them more pious. Maybe it does, but there are other factors involved.

For those of us looking at switching diets after our diagnosis, we'd like a little more information on the Mediterranean diet. But what little we have is conflicting.

Healthy volunteers show no change in colon cancer gut markers on the Mediterranean diet. But we do know that, in a test tube, extra virgin olive oil did slow down colon cancer cells. And the "olive oil and salad" model does lead to lower death overall in the elderly. So while a Mediterranean diet may not help, it might.

What about fiber? You've probably heard about the fiber wars, whether it helps prevent colon cancer. Some experts found no difference in colon cancer rates based on fiber intake. But other experts say eating high fiber foods prevents colon cancer. In smaller recent studies fiber did help but only for lower colon cancer (near the bottom end), and not necessarily for recurring cancers.

It turns out that lower colon cancer may be a different cancer than colon cancer of the upper or middle colon. Patients with upper or middle colon cancers have an overgrowth of biofilms, bacterial colonies that stay around and inflame the wall over time. Lower colon cancer patients get their irritation from the daily bacterial growth on the food you eat.

The type of fiber, as well as its size (how well you chew) affects what grows in your gut. There's so much new material about gut bacteria I wrote a separate book about it called *Tending Your Internal Garden*. Right now we don't know enough to say which bacteria are good or bad, because the bacteria can produce either cancer blocking or cancer growing chemicals depending on what's happening in the rest of the gut.

If you pay attention to the coffee studies, it turns out that coffee is good for colon cancer. But you'd better drink a lot. The protective effect of coffee shows up at about four cups a day! Before you start guzzling cups, coffee drinking lowered colon cancer but may have increased rectal cancer. So if you drink coffee, it seems to help. But if you don't drink coffee, I'm not sure it's a great idea to start.

There are a whole raft of other supplements you can take. Some of them may even help you (more on that later). But we don't know that they will.

A Summary of What To Eat

Less than two servings a week of red meat. Since frying, broiling and grilling are less than ideal, baked red meat seems to be the best. If you're going to have meat, make good local choices and find the best meat you can. We have no proof that this will help you, but it will help your community.

Less than two servings a day of refined flour. Basically get everything brown, not white. That is brown all the way through, not brown outside, white inside. Any brown grain will do, but look at things like quinoa (a grain that provides a whole protein).

Eat tons of fruits and vegetables every year. Yes, organic is likely to give you less pesticides up against your gut wall. And if the organic is more than twice as expensive you'll likely skimp on the vegetables. So get as many good vegetables as you can on your budget and remember every vegetable, organic or not, is better than that six-month old piece of dried meat they keep next to the cash register at the gas station.

Figure out how to get the sweetness in your life from whole fruits. Sugar is sugar, whether it comes from white powder, black molasses, brown maple syrup, or deep red agave. Slowing that sugar absorption by having it tied up in a whole fruit gives you a much slower body response.

Good oils are good for you. Olive oil, fish oil (from fish), coconut oil can help you make all those vegetables taste far better as well.

If someone asks you, tell them you eat the Mediterranean diet. There are many, many books out there to give you lots of guidance but focus on the idea of a full, homemade Italian meal with all the side dishes.

7 What To Eat On Chemo And Radiation

I haven't gone through your chemo or radiation protocol, so my information is academic, not personal. Take anything anyone who hasn't lived through it says about chemo with a very large grain of salt (or potassium).

When doctors do engage chemo and radiation patients in dietary discussions, it's usually about eating more calories. They are simply thinking about the myth that more calories in equals instant weight gain. If anyone of you has ever dieted, you know that doesn't work because fewer calories does not equal instant weight loss. When researchers tried this "eat more" dietary advice with colon cancer patients on chemo, they found that it didn't make any difference in survival. Upping your calories alone doesn't seem to help, so we need to do something different with diet.

But we don't even know for sure what to feed colon cancer patients when they aren't on chemotherapy. So we have to rely on "preliminary" studies on diet changes during chemotherapy, which means researchers still think that diet is too experimental a treatment to make broad recommendations during chemotherapy.

The first "preliminary" study I found was done back in 1995. A vegetarian diet with lots of fruits and vegetables slowed down the growth of cancer cells.

Twenty years later there's another "preliminary" study from 2015. It again found that vegetarian diets, with the possible addition of fish, might help prevent colon cancer.

So in the last twenty years have we done any diet studies on colon cancer patients in chemotherapy? Maybe even a Stage IV group where we know our standard options are poor? Nope. No major or minor studies that I could find.

We're just starting with the mouse trials, where they find – surprise- that a better diet helps the mice on chemo. Otherwise we have odd, single supplement trials like a Chinese trial that found feeding people on chemo helped them but giving colon cancer patients I.V. fish oil led to more complications (duh!).

Since one of the most common side effects of chemotherapy is nausea, maybe we'd find a study on which foods are less likely to cause nausea. But even those studies haven't been done.

When we try to piece together the individual ingredients of a possible diet, it still gets complicated. Individual ingredients might be helpful but we don't know how they act in combination. One of the most common assumptions is that eating more antioxidants during chemotherapy could be helpful, but just taking the antioxidants as pills doesn't give the same results as making them part of your daily diet. Just because meat products have many times less antioxidants than fruits, eating the fruits does not necessarily give you more benefit than simply avoiding the meat.

One study found no major benefit from adding antioxidants, with the possible exception of turmeric. Adding turmeric during radiation made cancer cells more responsive to the radiation. In a small study of advanced cancer patients, taking just turmeric may have some benefit in the gut but the turmeric wasn't absorbed well into the body to help with metastases.

Another food that might help during chemotherapy is onions, with one study comparing a high dose onion extract to chemotherapy and saying it was as effective as the current oral drug that is being used broadly for colon cancer chemotherapy

(Capecitabine/Xeloda). Saying onions might have a similar effect is pretty staggering. But more is not better. When given as 20% of the diet, onion extract made colon cancer grow in rats (and made them smell terrible). But a 5% onion diet blocked colon cancer in rats. Given that too much may make the cancer worse, we may be waiting a long time for the sauteed onion human trials.

One ingredient we know may help with cachexia (weight loss from cancer) is the amino acid glutamine. Glutamine lowers oxidation, slows cachexia, and nourishes the immune system and the gut lining. It's the preferred food of your gut lining, which normally has to feed itself from whatever you eat (rather than relying on your liver like the rest of your body).

One study estimated that a human patient recovering from surgery would need 0.2 grams of glutamine per kilogram of body weight to help. For those of us trapped by the English measuring system, 0.2 g/kg of glutamine is roughly half a gram per pound or 1.5 ounces of glutamine per one hundred pounds of body weight. That's a lot of glutamine, which doesn't have much taste but can get pretty messy as a powder. I'd do it in a smoothie if I was taking it, added last after all the other ingredients.

Other ingredients of an experimental chemo diet might include whey-hydrolyzed peptide, fermented milk, and isomaltulose. This combination was dubbed the immune moderating diet mix (IMD) and helped mice during chemo. It prevented weight loss without interfering with the chemotherapy.

When you're losing weight, remember that not all foods are equal. Anything made of protein or carbohydrate contains four calories. Anything made from fat contains nine calories. So if you're thinking about eating just a little bit, you can make a huge difference in calories by what you choose.

How many calories do you need on chemo? Let's start with how many calories you burn just lying around all day. It's called your resting metabolic rate, and there are calculators online that can tell you how many calories you burn while sleeping. For me, at 190 pounds, I burn 1784 calories a day just lying in bed.

If you're in late stage cancer, you have to add in the reality that your cancer is consuming a lot of calories as well because it's so active growing. So you probably need to add another five hundred calories to your resting metabolic rate just to keep from losing weight this week.

How do you get all those calories quickly without eating all day? Well, if you need fifteen hundred calories quickly, that's only about ¾ of a cup of fat. Cringe if you'd like, but anyone who's eaten lobster knows it's not uncommon to go through a cup of butter (mmm, butter).

To get the same fifteen hundred calories from protein or

carbohydrates you'd have to eat two cups of them. Remember that things like fruits and vegetables, while carbohydrates, are so full of good fiber that they don't count much in the calorie game. That's why they're so good for weight loss and not great for weight gain.

So, how do you get in ¾ of a cup of fat if you're trying to gain weight? Don't just drink oil because that is hard on the liver and gallbladder. Adding it to your cooking is the easiest way to get those added calories.

Here are some ideas:
Fish oil capsules (That's a lot of capsules).
Fish oil straight. One tablespoon is 122 calories.
Corn oil. One tablespoon is 122 calories.
Coconut oil/milk. One tablespoon is 117/34 calories.
Macadamia nuts. 204 calories an ounce.
Brazil nuts. 190 calories an ounce.
Sauteed mushrooms. 159 calories a cup.
Butter. 1,627 calories a cup. 102 calories a tablespoon.

Many people are using coconut oil at this point, which is a relatively quick way to get your calories. Be aware that coconut oil is saturated, so you may have some hardening of your arteries over the next decade. Not that we really care that much right now.

In addition to your fat, you want to stay as strong as possible. Mortality rates go up as strength decreases. Having the slowest walking speed of your fellow chemo patients almost triples your chances of dying. But how do you exercise when you're already exhausted from chemotherapy?

Here's a simple possible plan to discuss with your caregivers:

Every hour do 2 -5 minutes of resistance exercise (lifting yourself counts, whether you are standing up and sitting down or carefully climbing stairs).

Follow your exercise with a snack containing 150 calories: ¼ cup carbs or protein or 1 heaping tablespoon fat (a little over ½ ounce) That should get 1500 calories in throughout the day, assuming ten hours of waking time. Eat at mealtimes as well for extra calories.

What if you can't even move because you're too weak? Start tightening and releasing. This exercise routine is called Isometrics: movement without moving. It's the exercise routine of that icon of the old-time comic ads, Charles Atlas.

On a final, lighter note, an apple a day may keep the doctor away. But it takes two apples a day to keep colon cancer at bay. Seriously, Mice on apples had half as many gut precancerous changes. Researchers predicted that this would happen in humans who consume two apples per day.

8 Extreme Diets

Here's where it gets really interesting. Every day someone comes up with a new diet or supplement to "cure" cancer. Usually these "cures" come and go so fast you don't get any idea how well it might have worked over time. We need a diet that's been around long enough to judge if it has worked for people by curing their cancer for the rest of their lives.

In full disclosure, I'm on an extreme diet. My current diet is vegan (no animal anything), gluten-free (no wheat anything), and sugar-free (no added sugars of any kind). If you're wondering what I eat, it's plants and I may have fallen off the wagon by the time you read this book (update: not yet). So let's all be honest and say we really don't want me prescribing that to all of you. And I won't. It's my own deal, not yours.

But should you join me all the way down the extreme diet path and start drinking vegetable juice all day? Seriously, the Gerson Therapy requires up to thirteen fresh-pressed glasses a day. I'm picking on Gerson because it's well known, it's been around for over half a century, and because my family has experience with it.

So let's look at the Gerson Diet Therapy, which makes patients organic-only vegans as a start. If you switch to Gerson, you'll need a juicer and a lot of organic vegetables. All your meals will be plant-based, and you'll be drinking a fresh glass of organic vegetable juice up to every hour. That's in addition to your coffee enemas (up to five a day), as well as a range of supplements. The idea is that the vegetable juices provide you with easily absorbable nutrients, which helps the liver flush and the coffee enemas help the liver empty itself.

The good thing about Gerson is that it's been around forever, so we've got some long term follow up on people who've tried it. Back in 1958 Dr. Gerson said his dietary regime, followed to the letter (including drinking liver juice that they don't talk about anymore) could cure advanced cancer.

Fair enough, prove it. Gerson's program has lots of stories. I've even got one of my own. My grandfather went to Tijuana for the Gerson Cure after he was diagnosed with prostate cancer in the 1970s. He continued to eat a modified Gerson diet and occasionally juiced for the rest of his life. It worked because he lived to 102.

So why am I not racing out to get my fifty pounds of carrots for today's juicing? Well, we know now that prostate cancer can be incredibly slow growing. I'm not sure if granpa was cured or just long lasting because after his Gerson journey he didn't go to the regular doctors much.

We do have a study on skin cancer melanoma patients who did much better on Gerson Therapy than on regular treatments. The benefit for melanoma sounds right to me. In my own previous research I found that melanoma responds to carrot juice more than other cancers (the beta carotene color migrates to the skin, providing antioxidants and eventually making you orange).

But the Gerson Diet Therapy didn't do as well with pancreatic cancer. After a year of either Gerson Therapy or chemotherapy almost half the chemotherapy patients were still alive. Less than one in five of the Gerson Therapy patients survived the year. Yikes! That's not what we're looking to do!

So what do we know about colon cancer and the Gerson diet? Nothing. OK, there is one tiny study that says a Gerson-like program might help a little with metastatic colon cancer. But that's a lot of juice for maybe not much more benefit than just avoiding red meat and sugar. Yes, I know your friend-of-a-friend switched from rooting through dumpsters at the lard palace to hourly fresh-squeezed papaya juice baths and cured her colon cancer. It doesn't mean we should all do it.

Yes, after telling all of you to just avoid red meat and sugar I've gone way out there and decided to be a gluten-free, sugar-free vegan. If you just got that blank look, that's the normal response as your brain tries to process, "what can he eat?" Anything with plants, which includes things like potatoes, all the fruit I can eat, and every grain except wheat.

I came to my drastic diet decision through elimination and self-observance. Whenever I "sort of" have meat, I end up constantly eating meat. It's readily available, easy to cook, and never makes me feel that good. So cutting it out entirely is a lot less painful than trying to decide when I'm having it. I do have fish occasionally, but not weekly.

The gluten-free piece only comes because I found that wheat made me bleed out my rear. No wheat, almost no bleeding. So I kept that post-surgery because bleeding is not what I want to do. I don't have an immune response to wheat, so technically I'm not celiac. I just bleed when I eat wheat. No thanks. But for the rest of you, whole wheat may be protective (sorry, wheat haters). Especially red wheat.

Of all the bits of this new diet of mine, the no-sugar rule is the toughest. Check every salad dressing. Sugar added. So many things have sugar added in some way. I have to avoid most processed foods, and eating out is pretty sketchy.

But the no sugar rule comes from the scariest study I've found on cancer. It isn't colon cancer specific, so I don't know if it's applicable to you and yours. But it's scary enough that it's put me off all sugar.

The study was done by Colleen Huber. She does cancer support, and tracked her patients. These patients were doing conventional treatment as well as alternative treatments. As a result, their overall outcomes are better than someone doing straight conventional treatment. Even when her patients ate sugar, one third of them stayed in remission. But other patients avoided sugar, and almost half of them stayed in remission.

Remission is great, but what about survival rates? When Huber tracked her patients over time, about a third of them survived long term when they ate sugar. But if they avoided sugar their survival rate was more than doubled. Yes, that's enough to make me want to avoid all sugar for a long time to come.

What's the science behind avoiding sugar? We've known since the 1920's that cancer cells prefer sugar. They like to burn it even when other energy is available.

So, if cancer cells prefer sugar, why doesn't everyone with cancer just stop eating sugar? Unfortunately, many cancer cells give out signals to surrounding cells that they are injured and need help. That makes the cells around them their "zombie slaves" producing the energy the cancer cells need even if sugar isn't available. These cells surrounding the cancer will protect it from any efforts to kill it off by depriving it of sugar.

That's why the no sugar rule is what I'm doing rather than what all of you should do. All I can say for sure is that, while I can't starve my cancer cells by avoiding sugar, I can certainly make them less comfortable. You could go all the way non-sugar, but the only thing we can say for sure is that you should eat sugar sparingly.

9 Sugar And Biofilms

I mentioned a bit before how different parts of the colon might have different reasons for colon cancer. The upper and middle colon might have cancer caused by biofilms, while the lower colon develops cancer from wear-and-tear on the lining.

So what the heck is a biofilm? It's a little complicated. Before I got cancer I wrote a whole book called *Tending Your Internal Garden* about all the amazing things we're discovering in our guts including biofims. But I'll try to summarize the gut and biofilms here.

Basically, every one of us has far more bacteria in our guts than cells in our bodies. We're a hotel, or a walking rainforest.

Each one of us has a huge number of unique bacteria species (70% on average) inside us. We're pretty amazing.

What's more amazing is that these bacteria species don't just hang out on their own. They get together and form groups. Some of them get food, some of them make more little bacterias, and some of them protect the others. The way they protect themselves is by dumping out a gooey coating that keeps away any other species or any antibiotics. That coating and the species living inside it are called a biofilm.

Now, people with colon cancer have biofilms. People without colon cancer also have biofilms. But we're just starting to find out that some biofilms can be cancerous.

As I've been looking at the research over the past year, it seems like we've found one of the culprits for colon cancer, a bacteria that we know causes gum disease in the mouth. When it shows up in the gut as part of a biofilm, that biofilm can cause cancer. But it's not enough to just have that one bad bacteria, other bad bacteria need to come along and join it. A little like having a bad neighborhood, and having some really bad guys move in and make things worse.

So how do you stop the bad biofilms? Part of the problem is that any bacteria can go bad. Think about the innocent yogurt bacteria, lactobacillus. Totally harmless. Unless it becomes the dominant bacteria in your gut. Without competition, lactobacillus will start dumping out growth chemicals. These chemicals help the rest of the lactobacilli grow, but they also help cancer cells in our guts grow. Lactobacilli overgrowth can even increase cancer in the lower colon. Yikes!

So the trick is that you want diversity in your gut. Lots of different bacteria fighting it out, competing for space, so that no single group gets to dominate and start spitting out growth chemicals.

But sometimes we don't need the bacteria to spit out growth chemicals because we dump exactly what they need down on top of them. If you want one group of bacteria to grow, wipe out their competition with antibiotics then follow up with a lot of straight sugar that they can eat.

Mice fed a standard Western diet had their good bacteria start to go bad in a single day. We don't have the same studies on people, but we do know that diabetic people are at a higher risk of colon cancer.

So for those of us with colon cancer, straight sugar might not be the best choice, especially right after a round of antibiotics.

But things that will lower your sugar levels can be helpful. For diabetics, the drug Metformin has been shown to lower your risk of getting colon cancer. It's not likely that Metformin fights cancer, but it is likely that it decreases the overgrowth of sugar-loving, biofilm-making bacteria in your gut.

Whatever your diet was when you got colon cancer, you

THE COLON CANCER DIET

want to change it. Even if you think it was perfect. Why? Because whatever bacteria you had in there likely had learned to cooperate with colon cancer. Changing your diet shifts all the bacteria, which hopefully shifts your ongoing risk from those bacteria.

10 Supplements

Now we really speculate. Before you shell out for the newest supplement that cures colon cancer, let me sell you on one I like. This amazing supplement I'm thinking of has been used successfully without toxicity by millions of people. It blocks the cell growth in colon cancer cells, as well as blocking their migration through your body. Sometimes it even kills them off. Sound amazing?

How much would you pay for this cancer killer? How about four bucks in your local grocery store? Now available at the home shopping network: it's thyme. Yes, as in "Parsley, Sage, Rosemary and..." The effects of thyme on colon cancer increased with higher doses so maybe more is better, but we all realize that there is only so much thyme you can take on a given day before your stomach rebels.

I just used a test tube study of thyme to show that it's not that hard to do a study (unlike what many selling "miracle" supplements will say) and you can get some pretty definite results.

Whether the test tube thyme results apply to you as a colon cancer careful person isn't assured. (I prefer the term "careful" over the term "survivor" because "survivor" has a sort of gruesome, desperate quality.) But I'm very comfortable with thyme for long term use. Don't let your doctor get too concerned about supplement interactions with your treatments. Just ask if you can use "standard kitchen spices" in your meals.

Most of the known supplements for colon cancer can be added to your food in much larger quantities than you would reasonably get by swallowing them in capsules. If you don't like thyme as a spice, many other spice compounds block cancer cells in the test tube. The two spices I used in tablespoon quantities after my surgery to stop my bleeding quicker were turmeric and licorice. Both have the test tube effect of blocking the growth and migration of colon cancer cells, which is exactly what I wanted. Discuss the following with your doctors.

My Post-Surgery Repair mixture

8 oz water.

1 Tbsp turmeric powder (Banyan Botanicals)

1 Tbsp licorice (Banyan Botanicals)

Mix swiftly with a spoon and drink quickly or restir to keep the powder mixed in with the water. If it tastes terrible, you probably should try something else.

Other test tube studies have shown that cinnamon, pepper, garlic, and cumin all block colon cancer cells. So add more spice to your life by the teaspoon and the tablespoon. The only limits on spices is to avoid "burning" the gut with something like too much cayenne pepper, because inflammation helps cancer grow. Before anyone tells you test tube studies aren't applicable to humans, remember that our guts are basically one big test tube. We don't have to absorb the spice, we just need it to pass through.

But we do need to eat sufficient quantities of the spice to coat the lining. Imagine that I tried to get together enough capsules of turmeric and licorice to just swallow my tablespoons of spices rather than drinking them. A tablespoon of turmeric is equal to twelve grams of turmeric, or twenty-four standard capsules. Combine that with the same amount of licorice, and I'd be swallowing nearly a bottle's worth of capsules every day. But the same amount of spice as a tablespoon doesn't seem like that much, and I likely consumed twice that amount of turmeric every day in the weeks following my surgery.

While I strongly urge "eating" your supplements whenever possible, we do have one over-the-counter supplement that is fairly well researched. This common supplement really helped even those poor genetic Lynch Syndrome sufferers by decreasing the size of their polyps. It was so successful that all Lynch Syndrome patients are recommended to take it.

For the rest of us, this supplement decreased our risk of getting polyps after three years. It cut in half the estimated rate of death (mortality) among colon cancer patients who started taking it after their diagnosis. That's right, one supplement halved the rate of death of people like you and me. I think it should have been prescribed to me at my discharge from the hospital.

But I'm torn about starting this supplement for the simple reason that it is an acid and burns a small hole in your stomach every time you take it. That's a little blood, a little inflammation that might give me a false positive for blood in my stool. But looking again at the studies, I should take it myself. I think I'll try to find a source that isn't just going to sit and burn my stomach (Update: I chew ¼ of a standard tablet, which is bitter Follow up: it raised my CEA lab levels, so I stopped it again).

If you haven't guessed at this point, the supplement that halves our risk of dying from colon cancer is simple aspirin.

One a day, 325 mg, was what was used in the studies. Other studies found benefit from as little as 75 mg a day. For those who used it before their diagnosis, the benefit of using it after diagnosis was a thirty percent reduction in death.

For a proven colon cancer benefit, aspirin can't be beat. Just the benefit of adding aspirin alone should be worth whatever this book cost you. Discuss it with your doctors (you should be able to take it alongside any chemo or radiation).

The other supplement that is very hot right now, but doesn't have as much study, is vitamin D. Having the highest levels of vitamin D in your blood really lowers your mortality rates, by almost half again. But that study could be more about the overall lifestyle of people who take vitamin D rather than the vitamin D alone.

If you haven't had colon cancer more calcium might be an option as a supplement. Calcium showed less polyp growth, but had no effect in advanced colon cancer.

Before we go on, we have to talk about coffee again. Other caffeinated beverages and teas did not have the same effect. Several compounds in coffee block colon cancer growth. Some enterprising soul will likely isolate those compounds and market them as a cancer cure, but the evidence we have is for drinking coffee itself, in large amounts. Colon cancer patients drinking four or more cups a day had half the recurrence rate and half the death rate of colon cancer patients who had never drunk coffee. Now, I am not telling you to start drinking coffee. I will say that after a lifetime of avoiding it, I've tried it a few times. But I'm not really thinking about a lot of coffee until after I get my aspirin on board. (I drink half a cup a day now, combined with cocoa and chaga mushroom. Update: a year later I'm still on my crazy diet but no coffee.)

Supplements I take:

I do take the following supplements periodically. I have included the product codes for Emerson Ecologics, a doctor-only site. You can look up what I take and then order it elsewhere or get your doctor to order it for you. Emerson makes sure I don't get any heavy metals and my supplements are what they say they are on the label. I'm not affiliated with Emerson, I just use them.

Vitamin D (in olive oil, one drop = 2,000 IU) LIQ20 at Emerson.

Men's One a Day MOV40 at Emerson.

Modified Citrus Pectin 72060 at Emerson (I have powder, get capsules unless you don't mind doing smoothies because pectin makes your drink into a sugarless jam.)

A Probiotic SBC at Emerson. A member of the beer yeast family. (In my research I found that this probiotic lessens symptoms of ulcerative colitis in about half of patients.)

Turmeric TUR12 (I use the powder. Much cheaper but harder to take because of flavor and clumping.)

Licorice LIC26 at Emerson

Though I thought my vegan sugar-free binge would be short lived, I'm having more difficulty adding things to my diet than taking things away. My experiment with cold brewed coffee (three Tbsps coffee to three cups water, shake well and let stand overnight) hasn't really impressed me that much. I know the data is there for coffee, not tea. But it's just hard to get going on coffee after a lifetime of avoiding it.

The addition of aspirin is also hard to do, mostly because I don't want to have it burn a little hole in my stomach. So I chew it, which tastes terrible (it is an acid, after all. Salicylic acid). I haven't done this daily as I had intended.

I mention my own shortcomings so when you feel that "I'm not doing everything I could do" cancer patient guilt, you will know that you are not alone.

THE COLON CANCER EXERCISE PROGRAM

11 Does It Help With Colon Cancer?

Is it any surprise that exercise is helpful at preventing colon cancer? The lack of exercise alone is estimated to cause about one in every ten colon cancer cases. That's just from not exercising, forgetting about the increased risk of colon cancer from obesity. Our lack of exercise is so pronounced that researchers have been able to break down which lazy activities cause the most risk. They can tell us that watching lots of TV directly contributes to colon cancer in the U.S. (a little less than having a first degree relative diagnosed).

Don't get the idea that only a few studies support exercise for colon cancer prevention. The evidence is overwhelming. Experts reviewing three hundred different studies found convincing evidence across them all that colon cancer risk can be lowered by physical activity. Exercising more helps you die less often of colon cancer.

OK, maybe you're convinced that exercise might have prevented the colon cancer. It might help the rest of your family avoid it. But we've already got the colon cancer diagnosis. Will exercise work to help prevent recurrence in current cancer patients? Yes!

Looking at hundreds of women diagnosed with colon cancer, researchers found exercise very helpful. The women who exercised the most died at half the rate of women who did not. They didn't just die less of colon cancer, they died at half the rate from all causes. So women who got off their butts halved their risk of dying of colon cancer and, in a two-for-one special, also cut their chances in half of dying of anything else. There isn't a chemotherapy in the world that can give you those kinds of results.

I know all those fellas out there are saying, "that's for women. I'm a guy!" So let's look at a similar trial for men diagnosed with colon cancer. Men who exercised the most died at half the rate of those who exercised the least. And this wasn't just early colon cancers, this was early and late colon cancers.

Now, those of you who hate exercise are likely thinking those hot shots were all ironman triathletes. "Sure, great. If I could run a marathon I could lower my risk." But the bar for being a top athlete in the colon cancer Olympics is much, much lower. The top performers were walking an hour a day while the lowest performers, with twice the risk of dying, averaged less than an hour of walking a week.

So walking an hour a day for male colon cancer patients cut in half their risks of dying of colon cancer compared to those who walked one hour a week or less. Lace up those walking shoes!

Hopefully, you're convinced that diet and lifestyle might have something to do with your chances of colon cancer recurrence. Even if you aren't, remember that colon cancer patients are still at risk of other cancers and chronic diseases. So even if you don't change your diet and lifestyle to avoid the colon cancer recurrence, you want to do it for the rest of you.

The Colon Cancer Exercise Program:

Walk an hour a day.
That's it.

If that seems too easy, here's what I'm doing:

For surgical recovery, gentle stretching and deep breathing. The restriction on lifting after surgery is intended to avoid hernias, but a cough or sneeze puts far more pressure on our insides (they just can't tell us to never cough). Hernias happen when your intestines push out through the surgical cuts, so stronger and more flexible stomach muscles helps to prevent that.

Once you've been cleared by your surgeon, start swimming. Using a crawl stroke and kicking your legs will provide gentle strengthening to the stomach wall. Stretch, but don't tear! Stop if you feel anything painful and consult your surgeon.

Begin rebuilding your strength using small weights and building up. Six weeks of not lifting will have lowered your arm strength, so bring it back up to at least where you were before.

Create short exercise routines, which can be as simple as climbing up and down your stairs a few times. Find something fun to do, dancing, jumping rope, playing with children, to increase the times you breathe hard during the day. My own routine involves a jump rope and a chin up bar, both of which were hilarious to watch when I first started out.

Remember that the enemy of exercise is injury. Do not push yourself to pain, and stop if you feel pain. Always stretch your muscles before or after exercise, and honor their limits. Yes, this will really limit you when you're still recovering. But it's worth it to be able to maintain slowly rather than push harder than you can handle, tear something, and then fall off the exercise wagon.

Take up gentle movement classes, tai chi, hatha yoga, a walking program, or gentle dance. Explore what is available. Find exercise partners, people who will continue to motivate you.

If all of this sounds too complicated, remember it isn't necessary. All that is necessary is:

walk an hour a day.

12 Anaerobic Vs Aerobic Exercise?

Some of you will want more exercise advice, because walking just doesn't feel like enough. So let's talk about a larger exercise program for people diagnosed with colon cancer.

There are two schools of exercise. One group likes running, dancing, and thrashing about on a treadmill. These are the ones who breathe really heavily and think that aerobic (requiring oxygen or breathing) is the best kind of exercise. The other group likes lifting heavy things, grunting and straining. You can find them (outside of bathroom stalls) in weight rooms where they hold their breath and push large masses of metal around. These non-breathers are anerobic (no air) exercisers.

If you listen to either group, they've got true fitness all figured out. They are so sure of their own program that they tend to downplay the other group. The runners will talk down "bulking up," while the weight lifters will shake their heads at the stick-thin runners and tell you that's just not healthy.

So who's right, or is it really about a mix? The current fad is for high intensity workouts, which are shorter and supposedly better. But when you test people in all three settings, the results are the same. Starting a program of running (aerobic) vs. weightlifting (anaerobic) vs. sprinting (high intensity) won't make that much difference. All of them will make you stronger, and you'll get tired of doing them all within about three months. You'll likely get tired of sprinting even faster, and its intensity makes you more likely to injure yourself.

What about for colon cancer patients? Is it possible that, since cancer is anaerobic (doesn't need oxygen) that it prefers anaerobic exercise? Or does doing anaerobic exercise help the body fight the cancer?

So far, doctors have been so excited that their patients are exercising at all that they haven't done much research on which type of exercise helps. Either aerobic (walking) or anaerobic (lifting weights) helps cancer patients. Rat studies don't support one over the other.

The one thing that rat studies do support is not overdoing it. I should explain that rats don't exercise for fun. A rat study on exercise usually involves dropping the rat in water and making it swim for its life. When you do that, the rat exercises because it is very afraid it might drown. To increase the amount of exercise a rat does, the researchers strap weights to it while it swims. It turns out that adding a little weight to a swimming rat does make a difference in how many polyps the rat forms in its gut. It has fewer polyps than a rat who just sits around. But adding more weight doesn't help more. So there may be a "sweet spot" of exercise where you're helping your body and beyond which you're just hurting yourself.

As soon as you set down this book and go to the gym you'll likely hear something different. Brilliantly thoughtful advice will be given to you like, "no pain, no gain," or "just push through it," which somehow sounds convincing at the time. Never mind that the long term results of that kind of exercise mentality involve long periods of doing nothing while you recover from joint replacements.

Let me explain the most recent research on why you should aim for the "sweet spot" rather than exercising until your exhausted every day. When the body exercises, cells break down. There is literally a cost to pushing your body or a piece of iron across the floor, and it comes in the form of cells dying. Weight lifters are particularly excited by this process, because the body will use its resources to grown new, stronger cells in the old cells' place. These stronger cells are also bigger, giving a weight lifter bigger muscles.

That's right. Exercise sets up a situation in the body that supports the increased growth of rapidly dividing cells. If this sounds like a bad idea for colon cancer patients, it's because you're remembering that cancer cells are also rapidly dividing cells that we don't want to help grow.

It isn't just weight lifting that kills cells and promotes more new cell growth. Aerobic exercise also kills cells and promotes new cell growth. So aren't both of them a bad idea?

Yet we see in hundreds of studies that tell us exercise helps with cancer. So clearly something is happening that is a bit more complicated than simply cell breakdown and regrowth.

The most recent research explains the paradox. Exercise causes cell death. Cell death causes a short-term breakdown of the immune system as it is flooded with dead cells to clean up. But that immune system breakdown is followed by an immune system bounce back. The body releases lots more cleanup products. They speed up the collection of dead cells, increase the body's ability to fight infections, and decrease the inflammation in the surrounding area.

If you keep pushing the system beyond that "sweet spot" of the immune system rebound, you can overload the immune system. An overloaded immune system goes into emergency mode, producing lots of inflammation to marshal more blood and immune cells from other parts of the body. In other words, you just exercised to a point where you're making more inflammation than your body can handle. You are also helping your cancer, which loves inflammation as a trigger for more blood vessel growth to itself.

The process of cell breakdown can be seen in one kind of immune cell, a neutrophil. An active neutrophil pops open and creates a net with its own body to catch any stray bacteria and to help your body coagulate blood in case you cut yourself. Too many of these popping open at once, and you can get blood clots. We've all heard of the rare athlete who keels over from a sudden blood clot, likely caused in part by an overworked and overactive immune system.

For those of us looking at cancer, it's not just the clotting we worry about. If we overtax our system into chronic inflammation, we're helping rather than hurting our cancerous cells. Studies of colon cancers show that the cancer is more resistant to chronic inflammation than your normal gut cells. The normal cells will break down and die while the cancer thrives.

For those who advocate quick interval spurts or anaerobic weight training, the evidence just isn't there for weight lifting or quick interventions for cancer patients.

What we know is that moderate exercise, not extreme sports, will help colon cancer patients live longer. So we're back to walk an hour a day, and whatever else you'd like for fun without hurting yourself.

So is there a known "sweet spot" for how much we should exercise as cancer patients? We don't know for sure, but with the preliminary research we do have we can guess.

The point at which the body overcomes exercise inflammation and rebounds, which puts it into a heightened clean-up and repair mode, lies somewhere in the range of sixty to ninety minutes into the exercise. That's far longer than you'd get from either weight-lifting or interval training. The timing of heightened clean-up rebound didn't change much between non-exercisers and exercisers, which means it wasn't a training response but something that the body does for everyone. If you think about it for a minute, it should sound familiar. The best body response to exercise happens after about an hour, and that rebound continues for the next twenty-four hours as your body continues to clean up. In other words, walk for an hour a day (what am I, a broken record here?).

13 A Call For Research

Given how common colon cancer has become, it is hard to understand the continued lack of research in the area of diet and lifestyle for those of us who have been diagnosed. When you get a cancer diagnosis, you become very motivated to change what you can. Directing that motivation toward educated choices seems both wise and cost-effective. The worst thing that can be said of a positive change in diet and lifestyle is that it may not help avoid a colon cancer recurrence.

But few doctors would argue that an improved lifestyle won't help your risks of dying overall. Somehow the general advice doesn't apply to you once you've been diagnosed with colon cancer. It's this odd split between what will help everyone and what will specifically help those diagnosed with colon cancer that stops trials within colon cancer research centers.

In the past few years We're just now seeing the start of large studies on colon cancer patients and diet. Over the next five years we should have some better, more reliable information about what really helps. Look for the results of the COLON and CASUS colon cancer patient studies. Until then, we have to rely on what little research we have.

If you asked a doctor whether or not you should drink plenty of water after exercising, she would likely agree that hydrating after exercise is a good idea. But if you ask whether a diagnosed colon cancer patient should drink lots of water after exercising and you may get a warning that we have no "hard data" that tells us whether a colon cancer patient requires more fluids after exercise. You should probably discuss it with your oncologist.

In other words, a colon cancer patient has ceased to be a normal human being. We live in an artificial world where only the studies that start "colon cancer" apply to us.

Until we have more studies, my hope is that you've got what you needed to begin from this book. Just remember three things:

1) Rule 62 for weekly meat and daily carbs.

2) walk an hour a day

3) take aspirin if you can.

Thank you for reading and I wish you well on your journey.

Appendix: Recipes

One of the most interesting things about being on my crazy diet is that many people cannot believe it's possible. Remember, I'm not recommending this diet, but I know some of you will have questions about it. So let me lay out for you the diet of a man who no longer consumes wheat, anything animal, or anything with added sugar.

I'm not a chef, and I don't pretend to be. There are a number of very good vegan cookbooks which can be adapted to my "lifestyle choice." Take from this appendix only an idea of what you'd be signing up for if you decided to move to the far end of the diet spectrum. If you are more toward the middle, now's your chance to find one of the dozens of Mediterranean diet cookbooks and choose tonight's dinner.

For those who are still wanting to go on, we will.

If you want the two-second summary, I eat plants. But it gets a lot more complicated. When most of you eat plants, you coat it with a highly sugared dressing that makes it taste only as good as the dressing. A bit like eating cardboard chips with dressing on them. You're just eating the salad to get to the dressing.

I don't have the option of a store-bought dressing (seriously, all dressing seems to have sugar added). So I have vinegar and olive oil on my salads. And I have big salads, bread bowl sized, covered in hummus and avocado, because I need the fats.

Here's what I eat in an average week:

Four pounds of oatmeal.

Two pounds unsweetened coconut flakes.

Three pounds of mixed, frozen berries.

One pound of raisins.

One pound of walnuts.

Six pounds of rice.

Two pounds of red lentils.

One pound of beans.

One pound frozen broccoli.

One pound frozen mixed vegetables.

One pound hummus or chickpeas.

Four red onions.

½ pound of salad greens

One cucumber

Four avocados

One package cherry tomatoes.

One package tofu.

Sixteen tablespoons of turmeric.

Four tablespoons of licorice.

Five ounces of basil.

Five ounces of cilantro.

Substantial amounts of many other spices.

Aspirin. (1/2 standard 325mg tablet)

Coffee. (working up to two ½ cup a day, with one teaspoon cocoa and one teaspoon chaga mushroom).

So, what do I eat?

Not much fast food. I do eat the sofritas bowl at Chipotle, and eating Thai, Vietnamese, or Mexican food is much more likely to give you a lower sugar option. Still some sugar, but a lot less than standard American fare.

Here's a sample of my hard-core vegan, hold the sugar, hold the wheat, diet:

Breakfast

Oatmeal/Muesli
¼ cup sunflower seeds
¼ cup raisins
¼ cup coconut shreds
1½ cup oatmeal
½ cup frozen berries.

Bring three cups water to boil. Add sunflower seeds, raisins, and coconut shreds. Stir in oatmeal, then remove from heat immediately. Stir in frozen berries and let sit for five minutes to allow berries to thaw and flavor oatmeal. Serve sprinkled with cinnamon and nutmeg.

Lunch

Thai spring rolls

Rice spring roll wrapper
rice vermicelli noodles
handful cilantro
handful basil
bunch spring onions

tofu 1 block

spices

Break up tofu into small (crush it) pieces. Flavor with curry powder, garlic powder, pepper, and other spices to taste. Fry in olive oil on a cast iron skillet until starting to brown. Set aside to cool while prepared other things.

Boil water. Add rice vermicelli. Let simmer for three minutes, then take off the stove. Check periodically for softness and strain when soft. Place in bowl for making rolls.

Chop finely the basil, cilantro and green onions.

Dip the spring roll wrapper in hot water for ten seconds, then spread out on a damp plate for preparation.

Add a sprinkling of basil, cilantro, and green onions. Cover with vermicelli. Add one to two Tbsp of tofu mix. Bring sides up and roll as you would a burrito shell (bring the far side toward you, then lay over the closer side. Let the roll "set" for a few seconds to allow it to stick to itself). Serve with dipping sauce (Bragg's amino acids or a mustard).

Dinner

Rice and vegan sauce

Using a rice cooker, premake brown rice. Or, put brown rice in a pot with 2 ½ times the water as rice. Bring to a boil and simmer for ten minutes. Then let sit covered while you do everything else.

Red lentils 2 cups

Onions 1 large red

Spices to taste

Mixed frozen vegetables 1 pound

Frozen broccoli ½ pound

Boil water for the lentils (twice as much water as lentils). Add lentils and simmer for ten minutes.

In a big frying pan (preferably cast iron) mix up chopped onions and olive oil until the onions are limp. Then add frozen mixed vegetables and frozen broccoli. Cover. When the red lentils are done, add them and about a cup of their water to the onions and vegetables. Dump on spices (garlic and pepper, curry, anything that smells good). Cook together, adding water or uncovering as needed to get a good gravy consistency. Ladle over hot rice.

My standard salad is a big handful of mixed greens (as much as my hands can grab), which are to me the equivalent of the wrapping of a salad. Add eight cherry tomatoes, half a sliced cucumber, and half a sliced avocado. Then add four tablespoons of hummus, and a good glug (roughly four tablespoons) of balsamic vinegar. Sometimes I add olive oil, sometimes I leave it off. The goal is to have hummus or some other fat with every bite, so it never feels like it's going to be more work to chew the salad than I'll get in calories from the fat.

Fruit is your friend when you're sugar free. Fruit makes everything sweeter, and in a few days your taste buds will adapt. Frozen fruit smoothies replace sugar frozen treats.

ABOUT THE AUTHOR

Dr. Christopher Maloney, N.D., saw patients in family practice in Portland and Augusta Maine before finding out he had colon cancer. Since his diagnosis he's dedicated himself to spending more time with his family. He also changed his diet, exercises daily, and amazingly doesn't feel deprived.

Dr. Maloney hopes that each person reading his books will be helped. He can be reached at docmaloneynd@gmail.com. If you would like more information, including several chapters of the book that were edited out, please go to:

www.naturopathicmaine.com/coloncancerdiet.

Dr. Maloney cannot diagnose or treat your disease via the internet. He has hundreds of answers to common health questions at the blog Alternative Holistic Health Answers, as well as hundreds of answers as Christopher Maloney on Quora.

Post note: I also just published my thoughts on the spiritual aspect of this cancer journey, <u>Walking In The Valley Of The Shadow</u>, which deals with the fear and changes in relationships that cancer brings. While this book is about how to live with colon cancer, that book is exposing my soft underbelly to the world, talking about wrestling with death and my belief in God.

For more general subjects, I have other books, including <u>Tending Your Internal Garden</u> (the rainforest of bacteria in your gut) and <u>Your Car For Life: Basic Body Maintenance</u>. You can find them on Amazon or through Smashwords.

If you enjoyed this book, please review it at Amazon or elsewhere. Thanks for reading!

Made in United States
Troutdale, OR
11/18/2024